The Science of Mental Toughness

Raza Imam

Table of Contents

About Me

Like most 30-something guys with kids, I have a very busy life. Here's my typical day: An hour-long commute to and from work. Helping my 5 year-old with homework. Giving the kids baths. Putting them to bed. Doing dishes. Hanging out with the wife. And going to bed.

Not to mention the community service and volunteer work that I do, visiting friends and family on the weekends, and religious and spiritual commitments that I have.

Currently, I'm 36 with 3 kids, work a full-time job AND write books.

But it wasn't always like this for me.

For the longest time I wanted to make a side income, in addition to my full-time job.

I tried everything; "creative" real estate, internet marketing, blogging, starting a consulting business, and multi-level marketing.

But nothing ever stuck.

After a while, I learned about search engine optimization and created a fitness blog. It started seeing some success so I decided to take my diet and workouts seriously.

It took a few years to finally figure out how to eat and the exact right workouts to do, but after I got the information down, I started to focus.

So now that my fitness was where I wanted it to be, I decided to write a book. I called it "*The Science of Getting Ripped*":

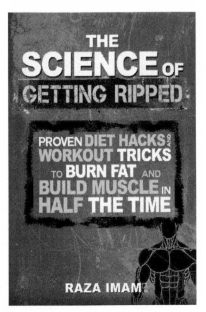

Click here to check it out

http://a.co/aTylaSr

I tried to market it and sell it, but then someone told me to put it on Amazon.

I focused hard on writing it, formatting it, publishing it and marketing it. After that, it became an Amazon best-seller in multiple categories.

Seeing these results was literally life-changing for me. I couldn't believe it.

It was all because I built the mental toughness to not only start and stick to a fitness program, but to push past my fears and doubts to actually write and publish a book about it.

My promise to you is to help you build a sense of mental toughness that helps you push past your discomfort, fear, anxiety, and certainty with a sense of dominance, confidence, power, authority, and mental toughness you never thought you could have.

I'll Help You Turbo-Charge Your Results

I really want to help you achieve your goals, and if you read this book and do the exercises for the next 30 days, I'm sure that you'll develop the focus and concentration you need to achieve your goals.

If you have a project that you need help with, email me at razasimam@outlook.com and I'll personally do what I can to help you get on track.

That's my personal email address and I give you permission to email me with your goals and what you need help with.

I want you to get the most out of this book and want to help you get focused so you can finally achieve your dreams.

Go ahead, email me now and I'll do my best to help you.

Here's my personal email again razasimam@outlook.com

(I do get a lot of emails and can't always reply right away)

Short and Sweet – No Fluff

"Give me a one-page bullet-list of exactly what I should do. That's worth more to me than a stack of books that I have to dig through to get to the good stuff. I may give you 50 bucks for the books. But I'll pay you $5,000 for the one page."

That's a quote from Alwyn Cosgrove, a world-famous strength coach and entrepreneur.

In this short book, I've shared simple, actionable, scientifically-proven exercises that you can perform to build mental toughness.

The best thing is that they only take a few minutes to complete.

This book is short, and that's for a reason.

I want to give you 100% actionable content, not a bunch of fluff and theory.

Sure, I give practical examples to prove my point.

Yes, I give you specific action items to do and I explain why.

Of course I tell you exactly how to implement these steps to get the best results.

But I worked *ruthlessly* to keep this book short and sweet.

So remember to take action!

So What Is Mental Toughness?

Before we start explaining strategies to help you develop mental toughness, we need to first explain exactly what mental toughness is.

So, it makes sense to spend the first chapter defining what we mean when we talk about mental toughness.

Simply put, mental toughness is the ability to look at hardship and adversity and *enjoy* it, knowing that you will eventually succeed.

To persevere through pain.

To keep going, despite defeat.

To push through heartbreak and disappointment.

To remain positive and expectant through obstacles.

To maintain a dominant, confident, authoritative attitude even though everything *looks* like it's going against you.

Mental toughness means looking beyond the current reality and acting with aggression, purpose, and determination to make your goal a reality.

It means to ignore naysayers.

It means to turn off the voice in your head that's telling you to quite.

It means to reject failure.

It means to embrace struggle, knowing that you will be victorious.

This is what separates the greatest scientists, philosophers, authors, business people, warriors, from their contemporaries.

It means to have an internal dialogue and remind yourself:

"I've got this, I love the challenge. This is easy and this is fun. I'm going to conquer this challenge. Hardship and difficulty make me stronger and I am going to succeed."

It means to train yourself to laugh at adversity.

It means to train yourself to push through discomfort.

It means to train yourself to view pain as pleasure.

Because after hardship comes ease.

That's mental toughness.

When faced with adversity and unexpected challenges, you smile at them and forge ahead rather than getting scared, worried, and anxious.

The Reality of Mental Toughness

Let's get real for a moment...

Sure, you can tell yourself that you love challenge and adversity and you can tell yourself that what you are doing does not really hurt.

But, in the end, if your body does not want to do something, can your mind really force your body to do something against its will?

The answer will surprise you.

For starters, consider the 2005 study that looked at the effects mental toughness had on male university sports students.

As the study notes, there was a significant connection between mental toughness and being able to hold a weight for longer.

Now, what does this study mean when it talks about mental toughness and how did it measure it?

Well, the study used a well-known questionnaire developed by researchers at a British university. The questionnaire is used to quantify mental toughness. Researchers identified 4 distinct components to mental toughness.

Those 4 components are:

- **Control:** A person who is mentally tough needs to be able to exercise control over their emotions and their life. People who have control of both will not get easily rattled, nor will they easily succumb to things like stress. They tend to be the people who you want around you in stressful situations as they can think clearly, even in the most hectic situations.

- **Confidence:** In order to have mental toughness, you need to be able to believe, deep down, that you are able to accomplish whatever you put your mind to. Some people do not attempt to run that extra mile or they do not attempt those extra ten reps because they do not think they can. But this is a massive issue. If you believe that you can't do something, then your body is going to follow along. If, on the other hand you believe deep down that you can accomplish something, then you will find that you can do it much easier.

- **Challenge:** Mentally tough people are not satisfied having things easy. They actively seek out new challenges so that they can conquer something new. Furthermore, mentally tough people are not disturbed by failure, rather they continue going, regardless of how many times they fail. Once they set themselves to completing a task or overcoming a challenge, they do not stop until they are done.

- **Commitment:** Essentially, mentally tough people are willing to work hard towards a goal and will sacrifice a lot of time and energy to see a goal through to its end. They will not stop until they are completely satisfied with the job they have done.

Let's look at a quote from a man who has proven himself to be truly mentally tough, Arnold Schwarzenegger.

From fitness, to business, to politics, Arnold Schwarzenegger learned how to overcome obstacles and achieve his goals.

In the 1977 documentary "Pumping Iron", Arnold says something that illustrates his attitude. He says:

"the last three or four reps is what makes the muscle grow. This area of pain divides the champion from someone else who is not a champion. That's what most

people lack, having the guts to go on and just say they'll go through the pain, no matter what happens."

This quote perfectly describes mental toughness.

It's an aggressive mindset that pushes you to take action, even though you don't want to.

So ask yourself, are you content with your life?

Have you ever wanted to build a business, write a book, get in shape, or learn a new language.

Do you often take up new hobbies, but then decide not to because it would require too much effort?

Do you want to start a new business in a new field, but are scared to do so because of the possibility of failure?

These are the sorts of questions you need to ask yourself and honestly answer if you want to determine whether you are mentally tough or not.

This book shares simple, scientific exercises that force you to push yourself out of your comfort zone so that you build mental toughness when it counts.

Master Your Breathing

Every human on earth is able to breathe, but very few truly understand the power that breathing holds.

Of course, everyone breathes normally, but learning how to control your breathing is a crucial part of mental toughness because during even the most stressful and hectic situations, deep breathing is a great way of getting control of yourself.

I'm sure most of you have seen movies or television shows where one character tells another character that is panicking to control themselves and breathe deeply. Now, obviously Hollywood has its fair share of inaccuracies, but this not one of them.

If you can master your breathing, you can easily master any stressful or hectic situation.

Let's take a closer look at deep breathing and how mastering it can help you greatly in life.

How To Perform Controlled Breathing

Before you can start doing controlled breathing and reaping the various benefits of it, you need to learn how to actually control your breathing.

In the 1970s, a man named Dr. Herbert Benson released a book titled *The Relaxation Response*, in which he detailed how to do controlled breathing. His book was one of the first English books on the topic and he helped introduce the effectiveness of controlled breathing to a western audience.

Like most things in life, controlled breathing is easy once you get the hang of it. It's comprised of 4 separate steps.

First, stop whatever you are doing and just focus on something in the distance or right in front of you.

Next, close your eyes and take a big inhale through your nose; make sure that when you inhale, you inhale deeply enough that you see your chest expand.

The next step involves holding that breath for 5 seconds. Make sure you do a nice, slow internal count.

The last step involves exhaling when you reach 5.

So, why exactly does this help you deal with stress?

Well, when you get into a very stressful or dangerous situation, your body activates what is called its "sympathetic nervous system." The sympathetic nervous system is responsible for our fight-or-flight system. Basically, when you get into a stressful situation, your body sort of loses its ability to think clearly and you go down to your base instincts.

Now, this an evolutionary trait that was very useful for survival once upon a time. But, nowadays, it just causes you to lose your ability to focus and think clearly when you need it the most.

Do you ever notice how so many people, who are otherwise very intelligent and clear thinkers, will make terrible decisions when they are stressed, put under pressure, or just in a very emotional situation? The reason for that is the stress is triggering their sympathetic nervous system, which impairs their ability to think clearly and focus on the issue at hand.

The deep breathing exercise above will trigger what is called your "parasympathetic nervous system." Whereas your sympathetic nervous system clouds your ability to think clearly, your parasympathetic nervous system will allow you to clear your head, focus on whatever it is you are doing, and think with a clear head.

Scientific study after scientific study has consistently backed up this idea and the studies have shown just how effective controlled breathing is at reducing stress.

For example, one study looked at the effects of controlled breathing on stress levels. This study took close to 40 healthy adults between the ages of 18 years old and 28 years old. It looked at salivary cortisol levels and heart rate and found that deep breathing sessions did have noticeable impacts on the stress levels of the people participating in the study. Both men and women equally benefited from the deep breathing sessions.

But, if that study does not convince you, there is a lot more evidence for the effectiveness of deep breathing.

For example, an by Dana Santas, a famous yoga instructor, goes into detail about why being able to control your breathing is important and why not knowing how to control your breathing can be very harmful to you. If you're wondering why her opinion is relevant, Santas has found success in the world of professional sports, where she has been the yoga trainer for numerous sports franchises across the MLB, the NBA, and the NHL. She has worked with teams like the Atlanta Braves, the Orlando Magic, and the Tampa Bay Lightning. So, clearly, there are many professional athletes out there who understand the importance of controlled breathing.

If all that is not enough to convince you, there is one more big example that shows just how effective controlled breathing is. Think of the most demanding, stressful, high-performance jobs in the world.

You'll probably think of world leaders, surgeons, trial lawyers, Wall Street executives, among others.

And you'd be right.

But the highest of all performers in the world are elite military units – their jobs are literally a matter of life or death.

Operators like Navy Seals and service members like the Marines are often put in high-intensity combat situations, where they and their comrades could get seriously injured or even die.

So, when the Navy Seals get into a stressful situation, what do you think they do to calm themselves down? If you guessed "controlled breathing," then you are 100% correct.

That's right, controlled breathing is effective at getting a hold of yourself and reducing stress, that it is used by people whose jobs often see them getting shot at.

I struggle to think of a more impressive endorsement than this. But of course, the Navy Seals did not invent this.

Those in combat have been using deep breathing for centuries. It has always been a well-known technique among warriors for reducing stress.

So, next time you get into a hectic or stressful situation, remember that breathing deeply when you're stressed, scared, angry, or anxious allows you to assume control of your body and physiological response so that you can think clearly, make decisions quickly, and ACT decisively.

The Science of "Active" Visualization

"It's hard to stay motivated during the tough training, but I just try to visualize myself on the starting line of the big race, and I know that I want to give my future self the gift of being as prepared as possible."

That is a powerful quote from American Olympic track star Nick Symmonds, who has participated in numerous events and won a silver medal at the World Championships in Athletics in 2013.

In this quote, you can see how Symmonds uses the idea of visualization to motivate himself during his training regimen (and anyone who has ever trained for an Olympic-level running event can tell you just how difficult and draining the training regimen is).

Your imagination is one of your most powerful motivators. Being able to create a mental image of future yourself succeeding is one of the best ways of motivating your current self to actually get up and work hard.

As you can see from the quote above, Symmonds has times where he wants to quit training and quit preparing for big races, but he motivates himself, not by focusing on his current situation, but by painting a mental image of what will happen after he has done all the hard work.

In this chapter we are going to look at the importance of visualization and painting mental images of your future success and how this will help you build up mental toughness.

What Is Visualization?

So, what do we mean when we talk about visualization?

Well, here's the thing, it is one thing to talk about achieving a goal. You can talk endlessly about how much you want something, how much you look forward to it, etc. But, at the end of the day, if you cannot sit down and see yourself doing something, then you will never achieve that.

By visualizing what it will be like when you finally accomplish whatever it is you want to accomplish, it will be much easier to achieve that particular goal.

For example, do you often do big projects at work that you avoid doing? Or school projects that you push off till the last minute? How about home improvement projects that you start but never finish because you're unmotivated?

If so, next time you are in the middle of a big project, try taking a few minutes to visualize how the great the project will look when it is done or how well it will be received when it is done.

Be sure to visualize the sense of pride and accomplishment you will feel when you are finally done. This is a fantastic method to motivate yourself to get through particularly difficult or draining periods.

Do you have a bunch of work to be finished, but you keep procrastinating because you don't feel like doing it and would rather push it off until another day? Well, try visualizing how much easier it will be if you were to just get the work done right now, as opposed to putting it off for another day.

But you can't just start out doing something and imagine what it would look like when you're done – that's daydreaming.

You need to visualize the steps in between.

This is what a lot of professional athletes do. For example, the New York Times wrote an article discussing how Olympic athletes use visualization to prepare themselves for big events.

Emily Cook, an American freestyle skier, had a very novel approach to visualization. She recorded herself laying out every single move and every single jump that she was going to make in an upcoming race; she made sure every possible detail was recorded. She then sat back closed her eyes, and played back the recording. This helped her visualize every little detail of the race. Cook ended up having the best performance of her career at the Sochi Olympics, and no doubt it was due in part to her novel use of visualization. But, she is hardly the only athlete to do so.

Plenty of Olympic athletes partake in visualization. That New York Times articles is full of quotes from various athletes who credit visualization as being one of their key strategies. If you look up any successful athlete, you will likely see that they engage in visualization.

Where's the Proof?

Now, we have presented a lot of good examples of visualization and how it can be useful, but you may be curious what science says about the matter.

Take a recent article in the Huffington Post by Srini Pillay, who is a noted psychiatrist and a professor of psychiatry at Harvard Medical School. He writes about how for years many scientists disregarded the power of visualization, dismissing it as a new age fad that had no real benefits and would soon fade away.

But researchers have begun to notice how powerful of a tool visualization is. When you visualize something, blood flows through your brain. A healthy flow of blood through your brain helps keep your brain healthy and it helps keep you focused. Dr. Pillay notes, much like we did in the earlier section, that athletes benefit from visualization as it helps them reduce their levels of stress and it helps them focus clearly on the task at hand. When the athletes are calmer, they make more decisive moves with more creativity and dynamism.

Dr. Pillay says that this same process of visualization can (and should) be used by business people and entrepreneurs, who undoubtedly face high levels of stress, anxiety, and worry in their professions. Visualizing the desired outcome and the steps you took to achieve it reduces the distress, allowing you to perform at your best.

So visualize yourself dominating your task. Visualize yourself taking control. Visualize yourself being triumphant. Visualize yourself as easily handling the task and plowing through obstacles.

Because rather than just visualizing a completed goal, you are going to visualize the steps necessary to achieve that goal – with a dominant mindset.

To illustrate this point, imagine what's going through Steph Curry's head when he was in the middle of the toughest game of his career against the Cleveland Cavaliers in 2016. What's going through his mind? What is he imagining? What is he thinking? How is he feeling? Exhausted? Absolutely. Nervous that they'll lose? Definitely. Stressed because he can't get the ball to do what he wants? Of course.

But I can bet you everytime he stepped onto the court he visualized himself as being dominant and successful. He visualized the plays he was going to run. He even visualized how the Cavs would respond to his plays.

And because the stakes were so high, he visualized them in a matter of seconds.

So, now you know the incredible power of visualization. If you haven't practiced visualization, or have struggled, the easiest way is to do the following:

1). Inhale deeply, hold your breath for 5 seconds, and then exhale slowly. Do this for 7 full breaths. Be deliberate, controlled, and purposeful with each breath. Visualize your breath coming in and out of your nostrils. It's helpful to imagine your breath as a steamy rainbow. Doing this will trigger your right brain (the creative side of your brain.)

2). Visualize that you're someone who is already successful and talk to yourself like them. Tell yourself "*I dominate. I know what I'm doing. I love this challenge. I know exactly how to respond and react. I do my best work under pressure and I'm going to succeed because I've worked hard and planned out every detail.*"

3). Visualize what you would be DOING to achieve that goal. For example, if you're preparing for a big job interview, imagine sitting confidently. Imagine answering questions using powerful stories, calmly conveying your confidence and expertise. Imagine the questions you would ask your future employers. Imagine how you would respond to trick questions. Visualize the entire interview with confidence, dominance, and authority.

In essence, visualization uses your imagination to paint a picture of how you will talk, think, feel, and ACT. We inadvertently spend so much time being stressed, worried, and scared, that we forget that we have the ability to visualize ourselves as strong, confident, and dominant – and ACT like it.

The Secret of Self-Talk

Jeffrey Immelt, the CEO of General Electric gave a talk at my company back in 2016. He painted a pretty grim picture...

GE's stock price was falling.

Officials in foreign countries that GE wanted to do business in were asking him for bribes (apparently that's how business gets done there)

GE had labor issues and unhappy employees.

Investors were upset and the struggling stock price.

He said despite all of that pressure, what allowed him to perform at the highest level is the ability to wake up every morning, look in the mirror and say, **"Hello handsome"** and keep on going.

That's the power of positive self-talk.

In the previous chapter, we talked about visualizing success and how it can help you. Positive self-talk is somewhat similar in concept to positive visualization.

With positive self-talk, your aim is to use words to pump yourself up and convince yourself that you are able to accomplish any task and overcome any challenge. It's often said that the subconscious mind can't tell the difference between fantasy and reality.

We have long known about the massive power of positive words. World leaders, generals, athletes, and other individuals in high-stress situations have always used positive words to pump themselves up and to pump up those around them.

Top athletes like Lebron James, Tiger Woods, and Tom Brady speak to themselves like the champions that they are. Military leaders speak to themselves as victors even before they step foot on the battlefield. Top business people and entrepreneurs view themselves as successful even when things are going well.

They are not deluding themselves.

Rather, they are speaking to themselves as the person that they want to become so that they raise the standard and take more action.

In other words, by speaking to themselves like champions, they are training themselves to ACT like champions.

History buffs and film buffs will no doubt be familiar with Patton's speech to the US 3rd Army shortly before they went into combat in WWII, which was brought to life on the big screen by veteran actor George C. Scott.

While the full speech is far too long to copy entirely, let's look at one particular passage that really illustrates what we mean when we talk about positive self-talk (you are heavily encouraged to read the full speech, it is easy to find and it is a great example of positive self-talk):

"Every single man in the Army plays a vital role. So don't ever let up. Don't ever think that your job is unimportant...No, thank God, Americans don't say that. Every man does his job. Every man is important."

As you can see here, there is no negativity in this speech. Patton does not denigrate anyone. He explains how everyone is important and that everyone can contribute. He is not the only general to do so either.

Military leaders for centuries have acknowledged just how important positivity is in their speeches. After all, men are unlikely to fight for you if you tell them that they have no hope of winning and that they are going to die.

So why would you speak to yourself any differently?

Never, talk down to yourself.

Never tell yourself that you cannot do something.

Never tell yourself that you're stupid.

Because self-talk sets internal expectations. And when you set low expectations, you get poor results.

For example, if you are dissatisfied with your current job and are thinking about starting your own business or moving into a new field, do not tell yourself that you cannot succeed. Always tell yourself that you can succeed at whatever you put your mind to.

The power of positive self-talk applies to more than just general's speeches. For example, there's a popular video of Elena Delle Donne, a WNBA superstar and former league MVP. In the video, Donne talks about how she uses positive language to really pump her teammates. She talks about how one game, a rookie was required to sub in for an injured veteran. The rookie was clearly nervous about starting their first game so soon.

Donne explains how she sat the rookie down and explained to them that they could succeed on the court. This positive talk ended really turning the game around for Donne's team. Donne also goes on to explain how she was shooting poorly and how she was talking negatively to herself, which only made her shoot worse.

Eventually, she began to talk positively to herself again, which resulted in her having a much better 2nd half.

She is not the only athlete to engage in positive self-talk either. If you look through the history of professional sports, it is full of great speeches given by coaches and players who truly understood just how effective positive small talk can be. If you do not believe her, there is more evidence to support what she says. Athletes have often reported that positive self-talk can help their performance and it can help them get through rough patches.

Before we talk about to how to engage in positive self-talk, let's look at one more example that really showcases the potential that positive self-talk has for helping people.

One looked at the effects positive self-talk had on people who had survived breast cancer. For those who are unaware, cancer survivors often suffer from a variety of issues due to the severity of the disease; these issues can include depression and severe stress.

Participants in the study received a personal, 2 hour long positive self-talk session and another 10-minute session conducted over the phone. Virtually all the participants confirmed that the positive self-talk sessions did significantly improve their ability to cope with their post-cancer stress and depression.

How to Engage in Positive Self-Talk

So, now that we have a fairly good idea of how effective positive self-talk is, how do you actually go about doing it? Is it as easy as just saying nice things to yourself? Well, here are 3 easy steps that you can follow that will allow you to engage in positive self-talk.

First off, you want to start by creating a few very positive phrases that you can say to yourself over and over again. The phrases should be relatively short, but also very powerful. So, for example, some good phrases would be things like

"I can do this,"

"I can succeed no matter what."

"I love the struggle"

"This is fun and this is easy"

"I'm going to make it happen"

"I dominate"

"I will figure this out"

You want something that you can continually say and that applies to as many situations as possible.

Secondly, get into the habit of saying your chosen phrase whenever you are in a situation that requires it. Just got assigned a bunch of work and are not sure if you can finish it on time?

Start talking positively.

Just started running and feeling like you want to give up?

Start talking positively.

Do not be afraid to tailor your phrases to the situation at hands. While you are running, you can modify your phrase by repeating to yourself "I am great at running," or "I can do this extra mile." After doing this for a while, it will soon become second nature to engage in positive self-talk.

Tell yourself that you enjoy the struggle. Tell yourself that hardship makes you stronger. Tell yourself that you learn from defeat. Tell yourself that disappointment only makes you better.

That's how you talk to yourself in difficult, trying, stressful circumstances.

By turning your pain into pleasure. By embracing the hardship. By, dare I say, *enjoying* it.

The Incredible Power of Purpose

Tony Robbins once said that human happiness can be summed up in one word – progress.

In this chapter, we are going to discuss the importance of getting a purpose in life.

When we say get a purpose, we mean that you need to figure out what your overarching goal is, either in life or at least in the long-term.

Because we gain true happiness when we make progress toward a worthy goal.

American President Ronald Reagan once said a very relevant quote that went like this:

"My philosophy of life is that if we make up our mind what we are going to make of our lives, then work hard towards that goal, we never lose, somehow we always win out in the end."

While Reagan is not the most uncontroversial figure of all time, even his biggest critics would be hard-pressed to disagree with him in this instance.

In life, you need a goal to work towards, an overarching purpose that you must achieve.

Having a purpose helps you push through periods of intense adversity. Think back to our chapter on visualization.

Remember how we talked about how being able to visualize your success can help you during tough moments or tasks? Well, being able to visualize your goal and being able to know that you are making progress towards that goal are amazing motivators.

For example, say your major goal is to lose a major amount of weight, like 50 or 100 pounds in a year. Obviously, in order to achieve that goal, you are going to have to exercise regularly. Somedays you may be tempted to throw in the towel and skip your exercising or cut your usual exercise session short. I know what you are saying, "I would never do that." A lot of people say that when they first start out doing something, but many times life simply gets in the way.

Being able to know that every mile you run or every pushup you do brings you one step closer to your goal is an amazing motivator. This chapter will focus primarily on two things:

First, we will show you how to set good goals for yourself through an easy, multi-step process.

Secondly, we will show you some evidence and some examples that demonstrate the importance of setting a purpose for yourself.

Set a Goal For Yourself

It is all well and good to talk about setting goals, but how should you actually go about setting a goal or a purpose?

When choosing a purpose in your life, go BIG. Like world-renowned rapper and lyricist Kanye West said:

"Shoot for the stars, so if you fall you land on a cloud"

Fighting world hunger.

Ending human trafficking.

Improving communication between struggling teens and their parents.

Creating the next billion dollar company.

Putting humans on Mars.

Helping couples on the verge of divorce.

Becoming the best piano player in the world.

Have HUGE life purpose. Or as Donald Trump would say "yuuuuge"

No one ever gets motivated by a small purpose. The bigger your purpose, the more motivated you'll be and the more support you'll be able to garner from others who are inspired by your passion.

But purpose and goals are two different things.

You can (and should) have a huge, ambitious, motivating, inspiring life purpose.

But you aren't going to solve world hunger in a year.

You aren't going to be the best piano player next month.

You will not inhabit Mars anytime soon.

These are worthy life purposes, but they are not achievable short-term goals.

It's important to remember this distinction.

You cannot pick a goal that is too ambitious, otherwise, you will not be able to accomplish it and you will not be able to motivate yourself by moving towards your goal.

Your goal should fit into your overarching life purpose, but it should be attainable and practical to achieve.

Here are the 5 guidelines that you should follow when setting a goal that aligns with your overall purpose:

- **Clarity:** The first thing you want to do when setting a goal for yourself is to make sure that it is a clear goal. For example, a goal to lose 100 pounds in a year is a very clear goal. Likewise, a goal to save up enough money to own your own home within 5 years is a very clear goal. On the other hand, a goal to just lose weight is not a clear goal. When it comes to setting goals, there should be no guessing game. It should be extremely clear what you want to accomplish.

- **Measurability**: When setting a goal, it is important that the goal is actually able to be measured. What I mean by this is that you cannot just set a goal that has no definitive end point. For example, say you make a goal to do 100 good deeds for people in a year. That goal is good because you can clearly measure your progress and know when you have completed the goal. If you just set generic, unmeasurable goals, you will not be able to look forward to completing them.

- **Time Limits**: When it comes to setting goals, time limits are important, they create a sense of urgency that will force you to continually make progress towards your goal. If you do not give yourself some sort of time limit, you also risk forgetting about your goals. After all, if there is no time limit, then it is very easy to procrastinate. Now, you do not need to give yourself a super strict time limit. Make sure you give yourself enough time to actually succeed at the goal.

- **Importance**: To put it simply, make sure that your goals are actually important. Make your goals revolve around things like your health, or your financial situation, or your personal life. Succeeding at goals takes a lot of effort, so you want to make sure that whatever goal you set is worth all that energy.

Having a LARGE purpose is so important because your short-term goals will need to align with it.

Does This Even Work?

You may be wondering whether goal setting actually works.

The answer is yes, yes it does.

In an interview with The Washington Post swimming coach Bruce Gemmell, who is the coach of American Olympic swimmer Katie Ledecky, he shares how important it was to create a big goal for her and to get her working towards it.

Professional athletes and their coaches recognize the value of setting ambitious goals. This is actually backed up by science as well. In one famous study, two researchers set out to find why there were big gaps in academic performance between people who were otherwise equally as smart (which was determined based on IQ tests). What the researchers found is that students with "grit" performed noticeably better than their peers.

Now, "grit" in this study refers to goal-oriented students. A student was considered to have "grit" if they had clear goals that they were willing to work towards. This study reveals that even if two people are equally as smart, those who have clear goals will just outperform those who do not have a purpose.

So set a big, ambitious purpose for your life. One that motivates you to push through the inevitable hardship, struggle, and pain you will face.

The Little-Known Science of Micro-Goals

Last chapter we talked about the usefulness of giving your life a purpose by establishing a goal that you want to work towards.

This chapter is going to build on the previous by discussing the usefulness of micro-goals.

See, the previous chapter focused on big, overarching goals (or big, fat, hairy goals as Olympic swimming coach Bruce Gemmell would describe them as), but this chapter will instead focus on the benefits of setting smaller, more manageable goals.

While big, overarching goals are useful, they can often take years to achieve which means that you have to wait a while before you actually get the satisfaction of completing your goals. Likewise, with big, open-ended goals you can oftentimes lose sight of the goal.

Setting small, manageable goals allows you to make progress towards a bigger goal, while still getting the satisfaction of actually completing a goal regularly.

In this chapter, we will be examining the power of micro-goals and why you should be setting them for yourself in addition to setting bigger goals for yourself.

How to Set a Micro-Goal

So, how do you go about setting a micro-goal for yourself? Well, the best thing to do is start with setting a big goal and then developing micro-goals that help you get closer to achieving your bigger goal.

For example, say you have a goal to write a 50,000 word book. Now, that is considered a big, overarching goal. It will likely take you quite a while to write a good book of that length.

Now, you want to create micro-goals based around that bigger goal. For example, try setting a micro-goal of writing at least 500-words a day. By setting a micro-goal of 500 words a day, you can feel satisfaction every time you reach that micro-goal.

Likewise, you will be able to feel intense satisfaction reaching that micro-goal because you know that each time you complete that micro-goal, that you are making more progress towards your bigger goal.

At a rate of 500 words a day, it will take 100 days to write a 50,000-word book. So, you make it a point to subtract one day from the total each time you meet your micro-goal.

Plus, by doing this, you can very easily get ahead of schedule, which always feels nice. For example, say one day you manage to write 1000-words instead of the usual 500, you can then sit back and say to yourself that you are ahead of schedule, which will give you a huge morale boost (be careful though, it can become very easy to procrastinate and quickly fall behind schedule).

You will also want to make sure that your micro-goals are actually small enough to be completed on a daily basis.

A lot of people already have experience setting micro-goals for themselves. Lots of people make use of "to-do lists," which, when you think about it, is really just a way of setting micro-goals for yourself. You have your bigger goal, which is to get all the housework done, you then proceed to break it into little micro-goals, which you then put on to a to-do list.

Why Micro-Goals Work

You may be wondering what it is about micro-goals that makes them so effective as a motivator? Well, the answer lies in how people react to achieving a goal. For example, noted athlete and trainer Christopher Bergland wrote an article in Psychology Today where he notes that achieving goals helps trigger positive chemical reactions in your brain which make you feel good. Likewise, Bergland also notes how giving yourself a small reward for completing a micro-goal can motivate you even more.

So, to go back to our book example, you could set it up so that after completing 500 words, you can watch an hour of television or do something else you enjoy. Doing this will give you the motivation you need to power through adversity and complete whatever it is you need to complete. Bergland is not the only who understands this either.

A very famous 2013 study looked at the effectiveness of micro-goals. The study took a group of people and offered them rewards in exchange for doing transcribing work.

The rewards were divided up into two bins. One group of people were allowed to take two rewards out of the same bin for completing their work, while another group was only allowed to take one reward out of a bin, they had to do another shift of work if they wanted to take another reward out of a different bin. The study found that those who only got one reward at a time worked harder and had more motivation than the group that got all the rewards at once. So, what does this study tell us? Simply put, the group that had one big, overarching goal (do the work and get all the rewards) worked less hard than the group that had multiple, smaller goals. This study presents a pretty powerful argument for the effectiveness of micro-goals.

Minda Zetlin, a noted author who has written several books on technology and the business world notes why micro-goals are so important for the business world. Setting micro-goals allows both management and regular employees to feel like they are really accomplishing things and making real progress.

Likewise, by focusing on micro-goals, businesses are better equipped to respond to sudden changes. In the volatile world of business, this is extremely important.

One last example is of US Navy SEALs and the notorious "Hell Week" they have to endure as part of their 6 month Basic Underwater Demolition training program. During "Hell Week", the trainees are put through 5-days of pushups, situps, runs on sandy beaches, obstacle courses (often with a 300 pound boat hoisted over their head) open water swims, and hours "surf torture" where they're forced to lay in the surf in the middle of the night —

during the course of the week, they are allowed *only 5 hours of sleep!*

80% of recruits drop out during hell week. Not just from the physical exhaustion, but from the mental exhaustion. Those that have been able to make it say they viewed it "one evolution at a time"

One 10 mile run until they get lunch.

Just one session of 500 pushups before they can close their eyes for 15 minutes.

Just 30 more minutes in the freezing cold water till they can warm up by the fire.

Just 2 more miles of the open ocean swim until they can get onto the boat.

The ones who were able to make it didn't look at making it through hell week. They just tried to make it through each "evolution".

So, by now you should understand the power of both big, overarching goals and smaller, manageable micro-goals. If you have not already started thinking about what micro-goals you can set for yourself, grab a pen and a piece of paper and start thinking about what you can do. One easy way to start would be by making a daily to-do list, which you will aim to complete every day. Eventually, you will want to develop micro-goals that help you get closer to achieving your bigger goals.

The Ancient Secret of Cold Showers

Up until now, we've discussed mental techniques you can use to build mental toughness. Things like breathing, visualization, self-talk, life purpose, and micro-goals. But starting from this chapter, we dive into practical, "physical" habits that will build mental toughness.

Likewise, people tend to take hot showers whenever they need to relax, which is usually what happens after a long, hard day. But, as you can probably tell from the chapter title, this chapter is not about hot showers, it is instead about the power of cold showers.

In this chapter, we will be going over the enormous benefits to be gained from replacing your hot showers, with cold showers.

Why Take Cold Showers

I haven't taken a warm shower in nearly a year... and I'm never looking back.

It's uncomfortable, *but that's exactly what you want*. You'll also notice an incredible sense of power and self-pride from taking cold showers. As you stand in the cold water, you're forced to control your breathing, to cope with the discomfort, and to eventually tell yourself that you love the challenge, you *enjoy* the challenge of the cold shower.

You'll feel powerful. You'll feel invincible. You'll feel proud of yourself for conquering your fear of discomfort. You'll feel dominant and confident because you rose to the challenge.

Just imagine starting your day like that.

Imagine carrying those feelings of pride, and confidence, and dominance, and power over to the other tasks you have to perform.

Studying for a tough exam – easy.

Making sales calls – piece of cake.

Negotiating a higher salary with your boss – no sweat.

You've started your day proving to yourself that you're powerful, you're determined, and you're mentally tough.

Eventually, you will not want to take anything besides cold showers.

Bottom line: taking cold showers helps you build up your mental toughness by forcing you to accept discomfort and to get used to it.

From a cosmetic standpoint, the use of cold water does not disrupt your skin's natural oils like hot water does. For example, famous model Miranda Kerr has credited cold showers with keeping her skin in good condition and helping keep her spirits up. She uses cold showers, yoga, and meditation to help keep her disciplined and strong.

Cold showers are also just very invigorating. If you are the type of person who struggles to get energy in the mornings, then cold showers will solve that problem easily. Plunging into cold water provides an exhilarating rush unmatched by anything else in the world. Katherine Hepburn, who was renowned for her self-discipline, took cold showers and described them as "exhilarating."

There is also scientific evidence that shows the benefits of cold showers. For example, a study looking at the effects of hydrotherapy (which is the process of using water to treat certain conditions), showed that taking cold showers helps increase your blood flow. The reason for this is that your body has to work overtime to keep your body's temperature at a normal level, which means that it has to increase blood flow. This is good for you because more blood flow leads to you feeling more energized. There is also some preliminary research out there that suggests that cold showers can potentially be used as a way of fighting depression. The idea behind this is that the cold water activates the body's sympathetic nervous system, which causes your body to release chemicals called endorphins, which improve your mood. More research is needed, but even still, it is a powerful argument in favor of cold showers.

How to Stomach a Cold Shower

So, how should you actually go about taking a cold shower? It is very easy to tell someone to take cold showers, but it is much harder to actually do that in reality. Stepping headfirst into a cold shower is an easy way to never want to take a cold shower again. So, let's go over the best way to ease yourself into a cold shower. Just follow these few easy steps and you will find that taking cold showers becomes much easier.

Get the Water Ice Cold Before Stepping Into the Shower

You might think that a good way to approach cold showers is to start off with a warm shower and very slowly start turning the temperature down. There are 2 reasons why this is a bad idea.

First off, it takes way too long. A lot of people only have 5-10 minutes to shower and doing this method will just take way too much time.

Secondly, by slowly turning down the temperature, you miss the initial, refreshing shock you get when you first take the plunge into an icy cold shower. So, just do yourself a favor and just go completely cold.

Go Feet First

Your feet are one of the parts of your body that adjusts to temperature changes most quickly. So, by going feet first, your feet will quickly get acclimated to the cold. So, angle the showerhead so that the cold water only hits your feet, then slowly move on from there.

Get Your Arms and Hands Wet

After your feet, your arms and hands are some of the best places to expose to the cold water because they also get used to the changes in temperatures very quickly. Plus, getting your hands and arms wet does not require you to move the showerhead at all, so it is the most logical step.

Plunge Your Head and Torso In

The next step is to get your head wet and to get your torso wet. This harder than the previous two because the torso and head are both very sensitive to temperature changes. So, the best strategy is to do what you would do in a cold lake, just plunge your head in. It will be shocking at first, but you will get used to it very quickly.

Get Your Back Wet

Now, the last part of your body that you need to get acclimated to the cold is your back. This is probably the toughest step (hence why it is last) since your back is very sensitive. Much like with your head and torso, you just need to get it done. So, turn your back to the showerhead and just very quickly back up and get your back soaked. Keep your back to the water for a few seconds or until your back acclimates to the cold.

Body Language of the Mentally Tough

Depending on how strict your parents or grandparents were when you were younger, you might remember being told to stop slouching and to correct your posture. However, emphasizing correct posture has fallen out of favor as evidenced by the fact that experts say 90% of Americans lean their necks forward when working, using the television, or using the computer, which is very poor posture.

The same experts also say that upwards of half of all Americans will complain about back pain in their lifetime, another sign of very poor posture. Now, when you were told to straighten up and to correct your posture, it was probably because people associate slouching with bad manners, but there are actually a lot of tangible benefits to good posture.

In this chapter, we will look at the surprising links between good posture and increased mood, increased productivity, and increased mental toughness.

What Does Science Say?

Many scientific studies have noted links between poor posture and feelings of things like depression, fatigue, and a feeling of inadequacy. On the other hand, good posture is linked with feelings of confidence, enthusiasm, and many other positive feelings. For example, in a 2015 study published in the very reputable journal, *Health Psychology*, researchers broke 74 people into two groups.

One group was told to sit with good posture, while the other was told to sit with bad posture. Both groups were given tape to hold them in place so that they could not change their posture. Both groups were then given identical tasks and tests, many of which involved reading and speaking. Likewise, they were also given physical tests, like mood tests and blood tests. The results are very telling.

Those with good posture were more enthusiastic, were less worried, were happier, and had a much higher sense of self-esteem.

On the other hand, those with negative posture scored poorly in those specific categories. People who had poor posture tended to use more negative language on both the speaking and writing tests. They also reported that they felt worse overall.

This is not the only scientific study to report on the benefits of good posture. Another 2014 study showed that having good posture can improve things like your perception and your ability to solve problems. So, not only does good posture make you feel better, it also improves your cognitive abilities as well.

Maintaining good posture is not just something scientists talk about either, both athletes and Hollywood stars understand the importance of posture. For actors and actresses, they are taught something called "the Alexander technique," which is designed to help them control their muscle movements while acting so that they can look more natural when on camera. A big part of the Alexander technique is maintaining good posture. Even megastar Hugh Jackman talks about the Alexander technique and the importance of good posture.

Athletes also recognize the immense value of good posture. Athletic performance consultants talk about how good posture can keep the muscles and bones healthy, which reduces the chances of injury.

How Does Good Posture Build Mental Toughness?

Now that you have a good idea of the importance of good posture and dominant body language, let's get back to the original topic of good posture and how it relates to mental toughness.

You may be wondering to yourself "how can posture and body language help me develop mental toughness?" Well for starters, as we saw in the previous section, good posture can make you feel more confident and positive.

When you are confident and positive, you feel like you can take on any challenge and you are far more likely to actually go out and challenge yourself.

On the other hand, those who maintained poor posture lacked self-esteem, which makes people timid and afraid to challenge themselves.

Powerful body language and posture changes how people perceive you. People do not like talking to people who slouch, it makes them think less of you subconsciously. If you have good posture, however, you're projecting the best image to other people, which will make you more confident when you interact with others – and it will make them respond to you with respect – in business situations and social life.

Imagine walking into a meeting boldly, confidently, with your chin up and chest out. Imagine sitting on the edge of your seat, leaning slightly forward, elbows on the table.

Or imagine being on a date and you sitting the same way – of course, making plenty of eye contact and sharing a warm, yet approving smile with your partner.

You will be taken seriously.

Amy Cuddy, a well-known expert on body language, spoke at length in a TED talk about how posture can define you, which is worth a watch for anyone who is interested in building mental toughness through good posture.

Powerful body language has been proven to change your blood chemistry, triggering the release of testosterone in your blood stream, and leading to feelings of confidence, pride, and dominance.

Not to dominate others, but to dominate your fears so that you take bold action.

So the next time you face a stressful situation like a sales call, job interview, difficult meeting with a client, go into a quiet room and stand tall, with your chin up and your chest out. Keep your legs slightly wider than shoulder width apart and just stand there. Imagine yourself as strong, confident, and dominant – as if you've just climbed a mountain and you're staring down at the landscape around you triumphantly.

Doing this for even 2 minutes will radically transform how you feel AND how you perform when you step into that difficult situation.

Here's How to Maintain Good Posture

So, like many of the things discussed so far in this book, maintaining good posture is easy in theory and difficult in reality. After all, if it was easy to do, more people would probably do it. So, here are some good tips for maintaining excellent posture.

Visualize Yourself Being Pulled Upwards

One simple way of maintaining proper posture is to visualize yourself being pulled upwards. Think about what you would look like if you were being pulled. If you are like most people, you would immediately go straight. Visualizing this can help you remember to correct your posture if you ever start slouching.

Associate an Object with Good Posture and Think About It Constantly

Another good tip would be to associate good posture with an object. Then, whenever you think about that object, you will remember to check your posture. Make it an object you think about often. Every time you think about that object, you will remember that you need to check your posture. After a while, it will become second nature.

Use a Mirror to Determine What Good Posture Looks Like

If you look online you will plenty of guides on how to maintain proper posture. The problem with these guides is that not everyone is built the same, which means that maintaining proper posture will require different instructions based on how the person is built. So, you should look in a mirror and try to achieve perfect posture, then make sure that you remember the steps you took to achieve that posture. You can then repeat the steps whenever you need to correct yourself.

Master Your Emotions

In this chapter, we are going to be looking at emotions and how keeping them under control is an essential part of mental toughness.

Sadness, hurt, anger, remorse, embarrassment, and fear are all human emotions that make us who we are. They are an inseparable part of us and denying them is unhealthy and destructive.

But, ACTING based on emotion is anything but healthy. Many situations in life require a firm head and clear thinking, which is not possible if you are letting your emotions rule you.

A common example of this would be if a family member ever got seriously injured. You need to be able to think clearly in that scenario and respond intelligently to the situation. Unfortunately, being ruled by emotion would cause fear, panic, and indecision – at the very moment that you most need to be poised, calm, and determined.

Dealing with fear, hurt, sadness, physical and emotional pain, and uncertainty requires a level of mental toughness that allows you to rise above the challenges of the current situation and take calm, confident action.

In difficult situations, you want to learn to harness those emotions and turn them into fuel, which you then use to motivate yourself to take action.

The Importance of Controlling Your Emotions

High-performers in all professions realize the importance of controlling their emotions.

Take for example the NBA and professional basketball players. Professional basketball players need to learn to control their emotions, otherwise, their game and their team will suffer. When players cannot control their emotions, they are prone to getting into fights with members of the other team, which results in fouls, suspensions, and fines (any basketball fan will remember the infamous fight between the Detroit Pistons and the Indiana Pacers).

Likewise, when players cannot control their emotions, they start missing shots that they normally would make. Famed NBA player Michael Jordan once talked about mastering his emotions before a game.

He explained how he gets nervous before games, but that he always made sure that he was completely calm once the game started by relying on his practice, his teammates, and his natural abilities. He put trust in himself, his coaches, his teammates, and his hard work during practice - and that helped instantly overcome the nervousness he felt.

Bo Hanson, an Australian Olympic rowing coach, talks about the importance of mastering your emotions. For athletes, mastering their emotions lets them turn it into fuel that they can use to reach peak performance. While Hanson is talking about from an athletic standpoint, there is nothing preventing you from doing the same.

Everyone has the potential to recognize the emotions they're feeling and them to drive themselves to do better at whatever it is they are doing.

To turn fear into ferocity.

To turn anxiety into determination.

To turn sadness into optimism.

You can't fight your emotions, doing so is a losing battle.

But you CAN learn to become comfortable with them – and with comfort comes control.

I'll show you how below...

How to Master Your Emotions

Mastering your emotions is not easy to do.

Anger, stress, sadness, and fear are all very powerful, and can trigger us to take actions that are unproductive at best, or destructive at worst.

Many of us are uncomfortable with our emotions.

We don't like to feel sad, so we may reach for the bottle to chase the sadness away.

We don't like to feel angry, so we may retaliate against the person that caused us hurt and anger.

We don't like to feel scared, so we do what we can to immediately seek comfort – which often means running away from our fears rather than facing them.

These are all instances of acting on emotion – and none of them are productive. They provide temporary relief to the problem. But action based on thought is what will lead to the correct solution.

The key to mastering your emotions is to learn to be comfortable with them... and then taking action based on clear and rationale thought.

This is called emotional intelligence.

Recognizing the emotions within yourself (and others), becoming comfortable with them, and then acting based on thought.

Here's how...

Do Something Relaxing

Doing something simple and relaxing is a great way of calming yourself down.

For example, taking a simple stroll around the park can actually reduce the amount of activity in your brain, which will help you keep your emotions firmly under control.

But, any calming activity can help you. Some people like to read. Others will do light exercise like jogging or yoga. It does not matter what activity you do to calm down, you should just do it.

Before making any decisions in an emotional situation, take an hour to do something to calm down and think on the matter. For example, are you being asked to make a very tough decision and you are worried about your emotions getting in the way?

Read a chapter from whatever you are reading, take a walk around the block, call a close friend, list out the pros and cons, and then make your decision.

Process How You're Feeling

One of my favorite ways to deal with emotion is to write down how I feel.

For example, if I'm stressed about work or some other life situation I create two columns: one for what's stressing me out. This is where I detail exactly how I feel. What I'm afraid of. The consequences I want to avoid. This allows me to process my fears, to become comfortable with them, and see them for what they are.

And then another column for solutions to my problems. Doing this allows me to make clear decisions after having already processed my emotions.

When I don't have time to document my feelings, I simply breathe deeply a few times, smile, and tell myself that I enjoy the discomfort of the situation.

Rather than fighting it, I learn to become comfortable with it, to see it as good for me. When I do that, my emotions seem to come under control, allowing me to make smarter, better decisions.

Understand the Purpose of Emotions

As I mentioned above, one of the keys to mastering your emotions is to understand them and become comfortable with them. You need to know why you feel those emotions, what triggers them, and how to respond to them productively.

For example, your body triggers anxiety because that helps you prepare for future threats. Your body triggers sadness when it is responding to a major loss.

Once you understand what triggers emotions, you can start to learn to counteract them.

Take anxiety; it is essentially a way for your body to tell you that you need to prepare for something.

So, by making sure you are properly prepared, you can master your anxiety.

Think back to school, did you ever notice how you could tell when you were truly prepared for an exam because you knew that you were truly prepared?

Another example could be the hurt and sadness caused by a bad breakup. The sadness and hurt may cloud your judgement, but thinking about it rationally could reveal that the relationship was not supportive and kind. And that despite the hurt that you're currently feeling, you'll be better off in the long run.

As Dr. Kevin Chapman says, emotions serve and adaptive purpose to help us survive and navigate the world around us.

So the key to mastering our emotions is to learn to be comfortable with them. To understand them. To use them to trigger thought that will lead to the correct action.

You will soon develop a reputation for being calm under pressure or for having "ice water in your veins"

Not because you don't feel emotion – but because despite feeling it, you don't let it rule you.

The Amazing Power of Black Coffee

Caffeine is one of the most widely consumed stimulants in the world. Over 80% of American adults consume coffee. When you consider that consumption rates are probably very similar all over the western world and indeed, the rest of the world, that works out to a lot of people drinking coffee.

Now, we all know why we drink coffee, it is a stimulant that helps give you that crucial boost of energy that you need to start your day just right. It also contains antioxidants, which provide a wide range of health benefits. It's a great pre-workout stimulant and a known appetite suppressant, which makes is great if you're looking to get into shape.

For most people, not being able to start their day with a piping hot cup of coffee is a good sign that the day is about to go horribly, horribly wrong. But, black coffee and the caffeine you get from it is not just a stimulant, it is a full-blown performance enhancer that will work to make every part of your body and mind work at peak efficiency.

Sure, black coffee does act as a stimulant, but unlike other caffeine based stimulants, like soda or energy drinks, black coffee helps you lose weight, think clearer, and just perform better all-around.

In this chapter we are going to explore the positive aspects of black coffee and why you should be incorporating a lot more black coffee into your diet.

Why Black?

But, before we get into the positive aspects of black coffee, let's address a question many of you no doubt are asking; why black coffee, as opposed to regular coffee with cream and sugar?

While it is true that those Frappuccinos and lattes that you get at Starbucks do have caffeine in them, it is not the same as plain, old black coffee.

See, regular coffee (especially if you have like many Americans do) and blended coffee drinks like the ones you get at Starbucks are loaded with sugar and dairy products like cream or milk.

The sugar and dairy products help counteract the positive effects of the caffeine. For example, caffeine helps give you a real boost of energy, but sugar gives you a sort of mild boost and then proceeds to essentially make your body crash; which massively impacts your performance, both mentally and physically.

Likewise, if you have even a mild lactose intolerance (like many people do), the dairy sits heavy on your stomach, which if you are trying to do something like exercise, will negatively impact your performance. So, do yourself a massive favor and skip the cream and sugar. Just go for regular black coffee.

I used to love the creamy, sugary, syrupy stuff, but have learned to appreciate a good cup of coffee. If you were like me, rest assured you'll be able to drink, and dare I say enjoy, black coffee.

Eventually, you will get used to the taste and as an added bonus, black coffee tends to be a lot cheaper than other coffee, so you will save a bit of money as well.

Benefits of Black Coffee

Black Coffee Improves Brain Function

Believe it or not, consumption of black coffee in moderate amounts can actually improve your brain function. In 2008 researchers reviewed 41 studies on caffeine and its effects on mood and cognitive performance as well as physical performance. They compared tea, instant coffee, ground coffee, hot chocolate, dark chocolate, and energy drinks.

And what it found confirmed what coffee drinkers have known forever... that caffeine and black coffee specifically boosts mood, improves cognitive function, and improved memory.

Just in general, studies like the one mentioned above show that black coffee and the caffeine it gives your body are good for cognitive functions. Now, you may be wondering how exactly that happens. We all know that caffeine gives you a boost of energy, but how does it actually go as far as to improve brain function.

You'll find the answer by looking at chemicals in your brain called "neurotransmitters." These chemicals are basically messengers that influence how your body and brain do certain things. There are two neurotransmitters called adenosine and benzodiazepine, which are essentially responsible for slowing down your body's cognitive functions. What black coffee does is essentially prevent these neurotransmitters from communicating with your brain. But, that is not all. Black coffee also enhances the effects of some other neurotransmitters which increase your brain's function, specifically dopamine, serotonin, and various other neurotransmitters. Because of all this, your brain is able to operate at a much higher rate of efficiency than it normally would.

Black Coffee Improves Athletic Performance

That's right, black coffee can improve your actual athletic performance. It does this by increasing the adrenaline levels in your body, which leads to your body being able to push itself that much harder when you do exercise, sports, weightlifting, or other physical activities.

Sarah Piampiano, a famous and decorated American triathlete, states that before any major bicycle race she will use black coffee to boost her performance levels. Plus, she isn't even a regular coffee user, she only drinks it a few times a year, but she still recognizes the value of coffee. She is one of the no doubt many athletes who use black coffee to improve their athletic performance before they step into the gym, onto the field, or into the arena.

I've lifted weights and worked out for a long time and I can tell you from personal experience, that drinking coffee before a workout does wonders for my performance in the gym. Science has even proven that it blunts pain so you feel less sore after your workout.

Black Coffee Helps Burn Fat

Caffeine is what is known in the diet world as a "thermogenic" This means that it is a stimulant capable of increasing your body's metabolic rate.

If you look up diet pills online, you will see that caffeine is an ingredient in almost every diet pill out there, the reason for this is because it is such a powerful thermogenic.

See, when your metabolic rate gets increased, your body starts to essentially burn fat at a far greater rate than it normally would. Because of this, black coffee can help you lose weight and burn fat without you lifting a single finger.

So, how does this help you achieve peak performance? Well, for starters getting rid of fat always make you feel better, which in turns helps you perform better. Also, increasing your metabolic rate can help you feel energized and thus better able to deal with whatever it is that you have to deal with.

Hopefully, you now understand all the major benefits of black coffee. So, next time you go out to Starbucks or your local coffee shop to get coffee, make sure you order it black instead of getting it loaded with dairy products and sugar; you will feel a lot better and you will also perform better as well.

The Secret of Waking Up Early

Most people have probably heard the little saying "early to bed early to rise." Slightly fewer people have probably heard the full quote, which is "early to bed early to rise makes a man healthy, wealthy, and wise." This fun little saying came to us courtesy of American founding father Benjamin Franklin.

Although Franklin said it best, he was hardly the only one to recognize the value of getting up early in the morning. A few years ago, Business Insider ran an article detailing the times that famous and successful people work up. Take a look at some of these names:

Marry Barry, CEO of General Motors is regularly in the office by 6am

Tim Armstrong, CEO of AOL wakes up between 5am and 5:15am

Ursula Burns, CEO of Xerox wakes up at 5:15am

Jeff Immelt, CEO of GE wakes up at 5:30am

Indra Nooyi, CEO of Pepsi wakes up at 4am

Bill Gross, PIMCO founder wakes up at 4:30am

Richard Branson, CEO of Virgin Group wakes up at 5:45am

Jack Dorsey, CEO of Square and co-founder of Twitter wakes up at 5:30am

Tim Cook, CEO of Apple wakes up at 3:45am

Bob Iger, CEO of Disney wakes up at 4:30

So clearly, many successful people wake up early in the morning. But, does the saying by Franklin have any truth? Does getting up early actually help you at all, or does it just result in your body being tired and you getting less sleep?

In this chapter, we are going to explore the importance of waking up early and how you can train your body so that you get up at the crack of dawn every day.

The Benefits of Waking Up Early

So, why should you sacrifice a few hours of sleep to get up earlier? There are actually a couple of very good reasons why you should get up earlier and we are going to explore them.

Visualize Your Day

If you have a family, particularly a very large one, then you know how difficult it can be to get a few quiet moments to yourself. Well, getting up early is a great way to make time to plan your day and visualize.

If you remember the previous chapter on visualization and breathing and were wondering when you'd have time to do it, well this is the time.

Waking up early gives you the peace and tranquility to breathe deeply and visualize your day. It gives you the opportunity to plan your day and imagine dominating your path. Using this time to strategize will pay dividends throughout your day. Be deliberate with your time, use the morning to plan how you're going to do that.

Time to Workout

One of the best reasons to get up early is that it allows you to fit in some early morning exercise. The biggest excuse for not working out is not having enough time. I get it, work, family, chores, social activities, etc. all take time. Those are are legitimate concerns, but waking up even 30 minutes early solves all of that.

Take your fitness seriously and be serious about it. Use this time early in the morning to get on it.

How To Get Up Early Consistently

It is very easy to say that you should get up early, but it is actually much harder to do so in reality. It is so easy and satisfying to just flop down and go back to bed when you first hear your alarm. So, here are some proven strategies that can help you get up early.

1) Have a Passion That Drives You

If you asked me to wake up at 5am everyday a few years ago I would have laughed at you...

But now, I do it everyday with enthusiasm, eagerness, and passion.

These days, I'm working HARD on building my coaching business, so I have to write, and write, and write to build up my audience.

Between my family and other responsibilities, I have to make time by waking up at 5am everyday.

Yes, I look forward to waking up at 5am.

Why? Because I have a goal that I'm passionate about.

You need to have something that you're insanely passionate about too.

I don't just mean work or school, because those are things you have to do.

You have to have something you want to do.

Maybe you want to start your own online business so that you can travel, maybe you want to

write a book so that you can finally fulfill your dream of becoming an author, or maybe you want to workout so you can get a 6-pack for the summer...

The actual reason does not matter.

What matters is that you have a goal that you desperately want to achieve.

Get into the mindset of thinking "every minute I spend with my head on the pillow is one less minute I can spend achieving my goal."

Trust me, once you get into this mindset, waking up early will be easy.

2) Go to Bed on Time

This is obvious, but it is also worth repeating, if you want to get up early, you need to get to bed early.

If you have a hard time going to bed on time you'll want to do a few things:

- **Be Careful About Naps**: Naps are a great way to boost your energy and productivity, but don't take naps longer than 30 minutes. Make sure that you take them early in the afternoons also

- **Have a Sleep Schedule**: Make sure you're getting at least six hours of sleep per night. Rather than wasting your nights binge watching "Better Call Saul", have a firm bed time in mind, and then plan your nightly activities around it. When it's time to go to bed, go to bed.

- **Create a Peaceful Sleeping Environment**: No electronics near the bed. A cool, quiet, dark room. A comfortable bed and pillow.Getting enough sleep is important. There's no use in waking up early if you're dead-tired all day long.

3) The Water "Trick"

I used to watch "The Simpsons" growing up and one episode that always stuck with me was when Bart drinks a ton of water so that he can wake up and open up his Christmas presents early.

As simple as this "trick" sounds, drinking a lot of water to wake up early actually works. In fact, drinking lots of water before bed was a strategy used by the Native Americans well into the 1900s.

It will take a few nights to find the optimal amount of water you need, so be prepared to spend a few nights tweaking your water intake until you finally wake up at your desired time.

For example, drinking 8 glasses of water before bed will just lead to you having wake up and go to the restroom in a couple of hours. Instead, drink 3 glasses of water before bed. If you find yourself waking up too early, (2am instead of 5am) you can should drink 2.5 glasses the following night. Keep lowering (or increasing) the amount of water that you drink each night until you finally figure out the optimal amount of water to wake you up I've used this trick and can say without a doubt, it works.

These are 3 great ways to help yourself wake up early and spend less time lounging around in bed. There are a bunch of great reasons to become an early riser, so do not put it off, try some of these tips and see if they help you become an early riser.

What Does Science Say?

Wondering if the idea of waking up early is backed up by science?

The answer is yes.

A 2012 study showed that rising early had positive effects on people's ability to remember important information and to do various tasks. Likewise, another 2007 showed that children who rose early had more energy and were more active than their peers who slept in.

So, it turns out that there is scientific backing for Franklin's saying about waking up early. Will getting up early necessarily make you wealthy? No. But, it definitely helps improve your productivity, and productivity is central to building wealth.

The Link Between Physical and Mental Toughness

For ages, people have known the link between physical health and mental health.

The Spartans.

The Romans.

The ancient Chinese.

Elite military personnel.

High-level business execs.

Physical exercise and mental clarity are inextricably linked.

But all too often people neglect to talk about the importance of mental health and the benefits that exercise can have when it comes to mental health.

So, rather than talk about the physical benefits of exercises like sprinting, weight lifting, walking, aerobics, etc., we are going to look at the mental benefits of exercise.

What Does Science Say?

So, let's first approach this from a scientific perspective. What does science say about the links between exercise and mental health?

Multiple studies from numerous countries have acknowledged the link that exists between mental health and exercise. This link exists in people of all ages, backgrounds, and professions.

For example, one study looked at the effects of exercise on school children. A couple dozen school children were broken up into 3 groups. One group sat for the entire time while working. Another group got one exercise session to break up the work. Finally, the last group got two exercise breaks. The results showed that the kids who got two exercise breaks did better across the board than those kids who got no exercise and those who only got one exercise session.

But, this phenomenon is not just linked to children either. Another study was done on groups of adults. In the study, participants were given a test that rates their creativity and ability to critically think. Participants were made to do the test sitting and then they were forced to retake the test after walking. The results showed that walking of all kinds (either on a treadmill or outside in the sun) resulted in participants doing much better on the tests. In fact, after doing some exercise, test scores went up by an amazing 81%.

So, what do both of these studies show us?

Well, for starters, they show us that even light exercise can drastically increase your ability to think critically and be creative.

Think about times in your life where you have struggled to figure out a solution to a problem. Did you notice how taking a walk and coming back to the problem made it much easier?

Now you know why.

The studies also show us that exercise in between work sessions can help make you more efficient.

The studies above looked at lighter exercises like walking and aerobics, but even more strenuous exercises like weight lifting and sprinting can be extremely helpful when it comes to mental health.

Some celebrities have even talked about how they use exercise to overcome their mental health issues and to make themselves mentally tough.

Famous actress Lena Dunham talked about she suffered from issues like depression and OCD. She found that medication did nothing for her, so she turned to exercise instead. The exercise helped her overcome her anxiety, depression, and OCD.

She isn't the only celebrity to credit exercise with helping them improve their mental toughness either. Khloe Kardashian, Ellie Goluding, and Oliva Munn, to name a few, all credit exercise with helping to make them mentally tough.

How Exactly Does it Help?

Physical activity clearly helps build mental toughness. But how?

What is it about physical exercise that actually makes you mentally stronger?

In the previous section we went over how exercise can increase your ability to think critically and how it can increase your creativity, so we will not mention that again, but you should remember that those are big advantages of regular exercise.

Improved Memory

That's right, physical exercise improves your ability to remember and recall information.

That's because when you get fitter your hippocampus actually grows. Now, this funny sounding word refers to the part of your brain that controls how you learn and you remember.

Gives a whole new meaning to the term "meathead", huh?

The focus, coordination, discipline, and perseverance required to workout further builds on your ability to stay calm, cool, and collected in tough situations.

In other words, doing a set of burpees, pushups, squats, or laps around a track despite the fatigue, "burn", or exhaustion you feel makes you more mentally tough.

Better Blood Flow

Another key reason that physical exercise is so useful for increasing your mental abilities is that physical exercise really gets your blood moving.

Your body needs to deliver more oxygen to parts of your body and thus it increases your blood flow.

A healthy, well nourished brain, full of oxygenated blood makes you smarter, sharper, and more calms. Obviously your muscles benefit from the increased blood flow and so does your brain.

Release Endorphins

This is truer for intense exercises like sprinting and weightlifting. Light exercise like walking and aerobics do not really increase endorphin production in the same way that sprinting and weight lifting does.

The endorphins released by your body help alleviate stress, tension, and anxiety. They give you a feeling of happiness and a feeling that you can really accomplish anything. If you have ever been seriously stressed out, then you know how difficult it can be to get anything done.

Like Ben Affleck's character in the classic movie "Boiler Room" said "motion creates emotion".

When you're feeling down, do something strenuous like calisthenics, weight training, running up stairs, sprinting on a track, or even something like chopping wood and notice how much more powerful, dominant, and unstoppable you feel.

Helps Fight Off Addiction

Whether it be to drugs, cigarettes, porn, alcohol, or any other sort of vice, addiction prevents you from reaching your true potential.

Intense exercise helps to distract your brain and prevent it from making your body crave whatever it is that you happen to be addicted to.

Also, the endorphins released when you train intensely helps placate your body and help keep your cravings manageable.

It's why so many runners report having a "runners high".

Or why weightlifters feel so powerful, resilient, and accomplished after an intense training session.

Addictions are hard to overcome, but working out can help overcome them.

So if you want to build mental toughness, be sure to test your body through intense physical activity. The feeling of accomplishment as you get stronger, leaner, faster, and more muscular will train you to deal with adversity and make you more mentally tough.

Direct Your Desire

In this chapter, we are going to change direction a bit and talk about something intensely personal, namely pornography and masturbation.

See, in the West, we often talk about various kinds of addictions, drug addictions, alcohol addictions, hell, we are even starting to talk about things like junk food addiction and video game addiction.

But, one thing you may not hear about often (probably due to the rather taboo subject nature), is the fact that many men in the West, and in American specifically, are addicted to pornography.

One showed that 77% of American men viewed porn at least once a month. Sure, many of those men maintain a healthy relationship with porn, but many others are addicted to porn and will consume it daily, which is very unhealthy.

So, in this chapter, we are going to be discussing porn addiction, why watching porn can be harmful, and the benefits to be gained by cutting back on your masturbation and porn watching.

This chapter is not just directed at those suffering from porn addiction either, it will also be very useful for anyone who watches porn and/or masturbates regularly.

Is Porn Addiction Real?

Some people may scoff at the idea that you can be addicted to porn, for some people you can only be addicted to things like cigarettes, alcohol, and drugs.

But, research has shown that things like porn, video games, etc., can have the same addictive qualities as narcotics and cigarettes. One study looks at the current literature published on porn addiction and concludes that yes, pornography can be considered addictive in the same way that any other vice can.

Watching pornography and masturbating releases endorphins throughout your body.

For a porn addict, watching pornography after not watching any porn for a few days would trigger the same sort of feeling that a smoker would get if they smoked a cigarette after not smoking for a few days.

Likewise, when a porn addict is denied access to pornography, they get the same sort of withdrawal symptoms that a smoker or drug addict would get.

Make no mistake about it, porn addiction is real and it is a growing problem in America and other places. However, due to the wide availability of porn, it is very difficult to actually overcome porn addiction.

Benefits of Cutting Down on Masturbation and Porn Addiction

But, not everyone is addicted to porn. In fact, many people who would consider themselves as having a healthy relationship with porn. So, why should these people cut down on their porn consumption and masturbation if they are not addicted? Well, everyone can take advantage of the benefits to be gained by cutting down on porn consumption and masturbation. Here are some of those benefits.

More Time for Other Things

This benefit applies a bit more to regular porn users than casual users, but it is still worth noting. Porn consumption takes up time that you could be using to do other, more productive things.

Now, you may be thinking that watching porn does not take up that much time, but time can fly by quickly when watching porn.

Plus, it is not just the watching, actually searching for the porn can waste quite a bit of time that would be better used elsewhere.

Better Sex Drive

Studies have shown that people uniformly prefer having sex with their partner as opposed to masturbating, but the two are not as disconnected as some people may think.

As numerous studies have showng (not to mention tons of anecdotal evidence) watching porn has a negative effect on a person's sex drive.

Likewise, studies have also shown that in many cases, when men are suffering from issues with their libido, cutting porn and masturbation out of their life alleviated their sexual issues.

So, even though everybody prefers having intercourse with their partner over masturbation, not many people seem to realize that their masturbation habits are actually making it harder for them to have sex with their partner.

Increased Testosterone Levels

One of the main purported benefits of stopping masturbation is that it helps increase your testosterone levels. Masturbating too much has been speculated to cause your testosterone levels to drop. Cutting out masturbation and pornography keeps your testosterone levels high so you can dominate your path.

High testosterone levels mean you'll have more energy, drive, resilience, and a healthy dose of aggression to channel into getting more fit, making more money, and overall improving your life.

Better Energy Levels

Masturbating takes up a good amount of energy. Likewise, once you actually finish, your body enters what is called a "refractory period," where it recuperates from its orgasm. During this period, you will have very little energy. Depending on the person, this refractory period can last for quite a while. By not masturbating and watching porn, you can save the energy that you would have used masturbating and apply it to other pursuits. Likewise, you can avoid the post-masturbation refractory period.

Of course, sex has this same refractory period, but the difference is that you're connecting with someone you love, building strong bonds, and even having a bio-chemical response from the endorphins that your body releases after passionate sex with a loved one.

Who Else Avoided Masturbation and Porn?

Now, you may be wondering who else out there actually avoided masturbation and pornography. Well, the list of people who did will surprise you.

For example, Apple CEO Steve Jobs was notorious both for his dislike of pornography and of orgasming, which he thought sapped his energy.

Likewise, there are many other famous people out there who forsook masturbation and pornography and choose to focus their energy elsewhere.

Miles Davis, a very famous Jazz musician, once said in an interview how he refused to masturbate or consume pornography because it sapped his energy, which he preferred to channel into his music. In fact, he was even taken to see a psychiatrist over his refusal to masturbate. The psychiatrist was shocked to hear that Davis did not masturbate.

Mental toughness is all about overcoming your base emotions and desires in order to reach peak performance. The problem with pornography and masturbation is that they represent us caving to those base emotions and desires.

If you want to build mental toughness, you need to have control over every aspect of your body and mind, and that includes your sex drive.

The Importance of Giving Freely

In this chapter, we are going to be looking at the power of giving, specifically charitable giving.

Have you ever wondered why so many rich, famous, and successful people give things to charity?

Sure, it helps their public image to be seen giving to charity, and for many, that is the case.

Yes, it's a tax-deductible write-off.

Yes, often times they create charitable foundations in their name like the George Lucas Educational Foundation, the Alec Baldwin Foundation, the Will and Jada Smith Family Foundation, and who could forget the scandal around Lance Armstrong and his LiveStrong foundation (Armstrong admitted to doping and LiveStrong has been accused of buffering Armstrong's public image)

But, that hardly explains why so many famous people (and regular people) give to charity, it also does not explain why successful people give so much.

If many of these celebrities were giving to charity solely to make themselves look good, then they would not be giving so much.

Consider people like Bill Gates and Warren Buffet, who are both known to give outrageous amounts of money to charity.

Bill Gates has already given close to $30 billion to charity, and he plans to eventually give away even more of his wealth in the near future.

The real reason why these celebrities give away such huge amounts to charity is that charitable giving actually has tangible benefits. In this chapter, we will look at the benefits of charitable giving and how it can aid you in developing mental toughness.

The Benefits of Charitable Giving

It Makes You Feel Better

One of the main benefits of giving to charity is that it just makes you feel better.

Numerous studies have documented the effect that charitable giving has on your mind and how it can make you feel better. This cuts across cultural barriers as well as age barriers.

For example, a 2012 study looked at the effect that charitable giving had on young people. The study found that when young people gave to charity they experienced a sudden surge of happiness. Even more telling is the fact that the study found that kids were happier when they had to actually give up something of their own. The study offered kids the chance to either give away something of their own to charity or just give something away while keeping their own stuff. It turns out that the children were happier when they choose to give away something of their own.

Another 2016 study from Sweden looked at the effects that charitable giving had on older adults. The study took a group of older adults and younger adults. They were asked to engage in charitable giving. After a few days, they were asked how they felt about the charitable giving.

While both groups said that they experienced positive feelings as a result of the charitable giving, the effect was more pronounced in the older adults. The study concluded by noting that while both groups get benefits from charitable giving, older adults experience even more benefit from the act. So, either way, this study further confirms that giving to charity just makes you feel better.

Giving to those less fortunate than you creates feelings of accomplishment, feeling needed, and a sense of pride. These feelings translate into resilience and mental toughness, helping it make harder, more difficult situations in life easier to tackle.

Gives You a Purpose

If you remember back to the early parts of this book, then you will recall that we talked about the importance of setting an overarching life goal for yourself. Well, if you are struggling to come up with a good overarching life goal, then you may want to consider some sort of charity based goal.

For example, pledging to give a certain amount to charity in a year is a great goal. You may also remember that we talked about the importance of micro-goals. Well, charity based micro-goals are also great options for those looking to set some micro-goals for themselves. You can set a micro-goal to help a certain amount of people per-day or set a micro-goal to give a certain amount of money each day.

No doubt a big reason why a lot of people devote their lives to charity is that it really does give you a great purpose in life.

For example, when I was a kid, my dad donated a gallon of blood over the course of a year (I still remember the key chain he got for it!) Now, he had to stay healthy and meet all of the medical requirements for giving blood, so it ended up benefitting his health too.

Improve Your Money Management Skills

One benefit of charitable giving that is not immediately apparent is the fact that charitable giving forces you to evaluate your finances and that it forces you to improve your ability to manage your finances.

If you set a goal to give $50 or $100 to charity every month, then you need to start finding ways to make sure that you can afford to give that money to charity every month. This may force you to evaluate your spending and figure out where you can cut wasteful spending. It may also force you to find creative ways of saving money, such as by cutting down on the amount of money you spend on things like groceries and gas.

It may even motivate you to look for a higher paying job, start a business, or start investing your money.

How Does It Help Build Mental Toughness?

Alright, so now that we have gone over some of the benefits of charitable giving, let's now move on to discussing how charitable giving can help build mental toughness.

The answer is not immediately obvious. Sure, charitable giving makes you feel good, but mental toughness is not just about feeling good.

By giving to charity you are essentially teaching your body to come to terms with losing possessions. You are training your subconscious to put less emphasis on material wealth like clothing, money, or whatever else you give to charity.

It is also a sign of self-confidence. When you give to charity, you are essentially saying to yourself that you do not mind giving away that money, because you know that you are successful enough to get it back shortly.

A big part of mental toughness is having self-confidence and regular charitable giving is a great way of building self-confidence. Of course, this is just covering charitable giving of money and possessions. If you go even further and actually volunteer to do things for charity (such as working at a soup kitchen), you are showing that you are responsible enough to balance your work life and your family life, all while finding time for charity.

All of this combined creates a sense of confidence, power, dominance, and self-determination that proves to yourself that you're a strong person and can handle deliberately giving because you know that you can get it back.

Destroy Excuses

This is one of the most powerful ways to build mental toughness. Yes, the other steps in this book are incredibly helpful, but taking responsibility for when things go wrong is what separates someone who talks the talk, and who actually walks the walk.

In this chapter, we are going to discuss excuses, more specifically, we are going to discuss why excuses are so bad and why you should avoid making them at all costs.

Making excuses is a universal human problem. Everyone makes mistakes and everyone tries to create excuses to stop themselves from taking the blame for the mistake.

From cheating spouses, to failing business leaders, to disgraced celebrities,   to minor fender bender accidents, everyone wants to place the blame somewhere else.

Excuse making is so ingrained into our culture and our being that it's pretty much second nature.

But if you are trying to build mental toughness, then making excuses for yourself is easily one of the worst things you can do. The reason is that it prevents you from improving.

When you make excuses for yourself, you don't feel the need to reflect, to assess, and ultimately improve. You can simply just make an excuse and move on.

In this chapter, I'm going to show you how to become "excuse proof". It's what former Navy SEAL Jocko Willink calls "extreme ownership" because when you take ownership for your failures, you can fix them.

Why Excuses Suck

Arnold Schwarzenegger has a funny video on YouTube where he talks about people who make excuses. One of Arnold's most telling quotes (and probably one of his best) is when he says *"if the president of the United States can find the time to work out, if the Pope can find time to work out, then you can find time to work out."*

Making excuses makes you a helpless victim.

In saying that, Schwarzenegger is responding to the people who make excuses to avoid doing something that they don't want to do, whether it's working out, or fulfilling a promise, or starting a business, or learning a new skill.

Consider this shocking statistic, on average, married men with full time jobs and children have approximately 3.5 hours of free time a day! And guess what they do with that time?

Watch t.v. (or Netflix or porn)

So when you say "I don't have time", you're actually saying "I'm not willing to make time".

For example, I have a job, and kids, and I take a class once a week, and I do consulting work for clients, and I'm writing this book.

I have VERY little free time, but I figured out a way to get this book written, keep my clients happy, spend time with my wife and kids, and grow my business.

How?

By waking up at 5am and working. By not watching t.v. By outsourcing menial tasks on sites like Fiverr.com. By leveraging relationships with friends that can help me.

I figure out a way to make the things that I want to happen.

Mental toughness is all about improving yourself so that you can unlock your true potential and reach peak efficiency.

This is why making excuses is so bad for your mental toughness. It prevents you from improving and makes you feel like a helpless victim.

The opposite of that is to feel powerful, dominant, resilient, unstoppable, and someone who makes things happen.

Which would you rather feel?

When you take charge and eliminate excuses, you feel a sense of power and self-confidence and control over your life that makes moving ahead so much easier.

It's almost like a high.

This is why deep breathing and visualization are so important. You want to get in the state of mind of feeling dominant and powerful and confident so that you can take responsibility for your actions and not let petty excuses and self pity sabotage your goals.

If you want scientific proof, there are a lot of studies out there that show that making excuses can be harmful to your performance.

For example, a study in the Journal of Psychology looked at students who make excuses in college and university. The study found that students who relied on excuses had a negative grade point average compared to those students who did not make excuses.

Science has also identified why people make excuses in the first place. In "Self Esteem: The Puzzle of Low Self-Regard" researchers discovered that people who make excuses excessively tend to be very low self-esteem people who are afraid of failure.

People with low self-esteem make excuses because they are scared of failure and think that by relying on excuses, they can avoid taking responsibility for their failure.

On the other hand, people with high self-esteem are not afraid of failure at all. The reason being that they know that everyone fails sometimes and that failure is a good chance to learn from your mistakes and grow as a person.

In fact, they view failure as a game, a challenge, a learning opportunity and adopt a "failure is not final" attitude.

This allows them to take responsibility for their failure, self-assess, and keep going.

How to STOP Making Excuses

Focus on How Mistakes Make You Grow

Many people make excuses because they see mistakes as negative things and want to distance themselves from the mistake by making excuses.

Ironically, one of the best things you can do for yourself is to stop treating mistakes as some massive negative thing.

Instead, whenever you make a mistake, immediately focus on how you can you use this to improve yourself and how this mistake can help you grow as a person. By doing this, you will turn mistakes from strictly negative experiences into positive ones, reducing the temptation to make excuses for yourself.

Adopting a playful, inquisitive attitude makes it much easier to accept the mistake and learn from it.

Focus on Larger Goals

A lot of the times, mistakes are small and mean little in the grand scheme of things.

A minor fender bender.

Paying a bill late.

Accidentally sending an email to the wrong person.

We've all done it.

But, we tend to take little mistakes to heart, which leads to them making excuses.

So, to avoid this, you should start focusing on your bigger goals. For example, next time you make a mistake, ask yourself "does this impact my ability to achieve my larger goals?" If the answer is no, then you do not need to worry about the mistake and you do not need to make excuses for it.

We talked very early on in the book about the importance of setting a big life goal, so this point ties in nicely with that one.

In fact, I once saw a speech by Jeff Immelt, the CEO of GE and he mentioned that despite the hardships he was facing as CEO, he had to wake up every morning, look in the mirror and say "Hello handsome" and figure out how he was going to run the company.

Get Used to Failure

It may sound self-defeating when talking about mental toughness, but you are going to have to learn to accept failure.

A lot of people go into things expecting that there will not be any bumps, and then when there are bumps, they start making excuses and give up.

Anytime you do something new, whether it be a new diet, a new exercise regimen, or a new business venture, tell yourself that there will be failures. Everyone fails, the important thing is that you own up to the failure and that you learn how to avoid it in the future.

As former Navy SEAL, best-selling author, and podcasting star Jocko Willink says *"all your excuses are lies"*

Assess Your Appetite

In this last chapter, we are going to discuss a prevalent problem in America, namely the problem of mindless eating.

In 2006, Cornell professor Brian Wansink published a book called "Mindless Eating: Why We Eat More Than We Think We Do". In the book, he explored why Americans eat as much as they do. A big idea he talked in the book was the idea of "mindless eating," which basically refers to the fact that many people mindlessly eat based on subconscious factors such as packaging, product names, containers, etc.

Basically, Americans (and those in other western countries) eat too much because a variety of factors subconsciously influence them to eat unhealthy foods.

If you want to be mentally tough, you have to learn to consciously control your actions. So, this chapter is going to focus on how you can escape the scourge of mindless eating.

Mindless Eating?

So, in the intro, I briefly touched on what mindless eating is, but in this section, I'm going to give a bit more information about mindless eating before covering how you can avoid it - so you become a mentally tough badass.

Have you ever noticed that when you sit down to watch television, you naturally gravitate towards eating junk food? Likewise, have you ever noticed that when shopping for stuff, you seem to gravitate towards brightly colored packaging? Or how you're subconsciously primed to buy the jumbo bucket of popcorn at the movies?

Mindless eating... all of it.

Are you actually hungry?

Are you paying attention to how the food actually tastes?

Do you notice how eating that stuff makes you feel?

Do you even like popcorn???

Important questions to ask yourself when you find yourself stuffing your face for no good reason.

Believe it or not, a major reason for overeating is pure boredom.

For some reason, we are conditioned to think about eating when we get bored, even if we aren't particularly hungry.

This topic was the subject of a very interesting study done in 2015. There were three separate studies done as part of this one big study.

The first study asked the participants to keep a diary in which they tracked their boredom levels and their food intake. After a week, the diaries showed that on days when the boredom level was higher, the intake of high calorie, high-fat foods also increased.

The second study also showed something very similar. In this study, participants were asked to do a task that was very boring and one that was less boring. When doing the very boring task, the desire to eat snacks, particularly unhealthy snacks, skyrocketed.

Finally, the third study essentially replicated the second one and again showed that when doing something very boring, the desire to eat sugary, high-fat junk food massively increases. The third study also showed that when doing something boring, the desire to eat healthy, unexciting foods like cut up veggies did not increase.

On top of eating when we're bored, we eat when we're stressed. Hence the term emotional eating.

Like an ostrich sticking its head in the sand, eating when we're stressed, bored, or excited won't make life more exciting and definitely won't make our problems disappear.

Alright, so now that we have a better idea of what mindless eating is, how should you go about avoiding it?

After all, if so much of mindless eating is made up of subconscious factors, then surely it must be difficult to do. I am not going to lie and tell you that overcoming mindless eating is easy because it is not, but it is certainly possible. Besides, nothing about mental toughness is easy, if developing mental toughness was easy everyone would do it.

So, here are some strategies you can use to break your mindless eating habit.

Our relationship with food is complex and diverse, and I'm not going to psychoanalyze why (not that I even could)

What I WILL do is show you how to be mentally tough by controlling your urge to put food in your mouth when you don't need (or even truly want) to.

Eat Your Favorite Foods, But Pre-Plan Your Meals

Buying stuff makes us feel good. New clothes, new gadgets, new jewelry, new cars.

But you don't waltz into the car dealership and buy the first car that excites you.

You don't walk into the jewelry store and buy the first piece of jewelry that catches your eye.

And no matter how much of a fanboy (or girl) you are, you don't go to the Apple store and buy every single Apple product you see (or do you???)

You walk into the store with a budget and you stick to it.

But for some reason, we feel comfortable stuffing our faces with whatever we feel like, because it makes us feel good.

So if you want to control what you eat, you have to make a list of your favorite foods.

Mine are french toast, buffalo chicken, peanut butter and jelly, chocolate almonds, mangos, blueberries, broccoli, ground turkey, taco salad.

Just thinking about those foods makes me happy.

Now that I have a list of my favorite foods, I pre-plan my meals so they're ready to go for the week.

When I have time, I'll grill some chicken breasts with buffalo sauce and make some broccoli afterwards.

At the same time, I'll saute some ground turkey for taco salad.

I'll buy greek yogurt and add blueberries and chocolate almonds to it.

The key is that I do measure my foods and make sure that I'm eating the right amount of calories for my needs (more on days that I lift weights, and less on days that I don't)

This way, I'm still eating my absolute favorite foods, which helps me not binge on junk.

This is how professional models, actors, and bodybuilders eat - and it helps them get in great shape. By using prepared meals, you avoid keeping any snacks in your home, which makes it basically impossible to mindlessly grab unhealthy snacks.

Jordin Sparks, an American singer who is most famous for winning season 6 of American Idol, credits her weight loss with the fact that she used prepared meals, which helped her cut down on unnecessary snacking.

Just pick a day (most people choose Sunday, but pick whatever works for you) and buy all the ingredients you need to make your prepared meals for the rest of the week.

Don't Be Idle

The thing about mindless snacking is that it happens most often when you are bored; this was demonstrated in the studies I mentioned earlier.

A good strategy for avoiding mindless eating is to avoid getting bored.

The best option is to develop the habit of working out, even if it's just for 30 seconds.

If you're working at your computer and feel the urge to grab a bag of chips, get on the floor and do 10 pushups. Or 10 jumping jacks. Or 10 squats.

Trust me, you'll feel accomplished and proud of yourself. This sense of pride and accomplishment will help subside your cravings and crush your boredom.

You'll feel a sense of control and mental toughness that will propel you through your day.

Drink More Fluids

Often times, we eat because we're actually thirsty.

So rather than grabbing a cookie, grab a glass of water.

If you're feeling slightly hungry, drink a cup of black coffee. I mentioned the benefits of drinking coffee in a previous chapter, but I'll say it again. Drinking coffee helps reduce hunger.

Get More Sleep

One last item to mention is sleep. When we don't get enough sleep, we lose all of our self-control... especially when it comes to eating.

There was a famous study done at the University of Chicago about this.

People on 5.5h of sleep lost 55% less fat and lost A LOT more muscle than people on 8h of sleep.

Why? Low sleep messes with your hormones.

Sleep-deprivation will lower your leptin while spiking ghrelin and cortisol. Very broadly speaking, this means you will have more food cravings, will feel less overall satiety, and experience way more stress.

Lack of sleep kills your self-control

Another study showed that sleep deprivation decreases the activity of your prefrontal cortex. Meaning you will have less willpower and self-control, which surely won't help when you're trying to resist that tempting muffin.

So if you want to be mentally tough, you have to stop mindless eating.

Bonus: Mental Toughness Meditation

One of the best self-help books of all time is Psycho-Cybernetics written by Dr. Maxwell Maltz in the 1960's. He was a plastic surgeon that noticed patients who have had their limbs amputated still felt pain that limb.

Even though it had been amputated.

This got him thinking about self-image. He concluded that we become what we think about. He's not the first one to say this, but it really resonated with me.

The whole point of his book is that your mind is like a "heat seeking missile" If it has a goal, infused with emotion and passion, it will figure out how to accomplish it.

There will be trial and error, but if you keep believing in your goal and take action, you will eventually achieve it. He gives the example of a baby reaching for an object on a table. When he first reaches for it, he might miss, but he will eventually get it.

So belief creates a positive self-image. When you create a positive self-image of yourself ALREADY having accomplished your goal, you will have the motivation and drive to figure out it.

Here's a brief meditation you can try:

Sit back, openly, confidently, and expectantly with your arms at your side and your head leaning back slightly.

Close your eyes and smile ever so slightly with your mouth and jaws loose and relaxed.

Imagine you're sitting on a cruise ship, looking out at a dark sky early in the morning. The horizon looks purple and is almost glowing. As you sit there, imagine a warm golden rain falling gently on your body.

Enjoy the beautiful peace, and warmth, and serenity of this powerful scene.

Now imagine the goal that you seek to achieve. ***Imagine yourself already having achieved it.***

Imagine the power, and confidence, and excitement, and enthusiasm, and gratitude you would feel once you're accomplished it.

KNOW in your mind that you've already achieved it.

Now, imagine the steps you took to make it a reality.

Imagine how you acted.

Imagine what you did.

Imagine the obstacles you faced and how you overcame them.

Imagine that you're someone else if you have to and view the world through their eyes.

Talk to yourself like them.

Think like them.

Imagine acting like them.

Know that this is the secret to achieving your goals is **to build the mindset and take actions of someone that is already successful.**

Feel it.
Believe it.
Expect it.

Doing this meditation for 5 minutes every day will mold your subconscious mind to expect that reality. It will sharpen your focus, enhance your motivation, and help guide you to the actions and activities that you need to take to achieve them.

It's incredibly powerful.

Now go do it and enjoy the feelings of pride, confidence, gratitude, and excitement that come with it.

1). So choose a goal.

2). Imagine, visualize, and see yourself having already achieved it.

3). Sense the amazing feelings of achieving your goal.

4). Use the steps in this book to build focus so that you can create it in reality.

Here's What To Do Next

I hope you enjoyed this book.

But more than that I hope that you take action.

Things don't happen by themselves and you're the only one that's responsible for your situation in life.

If you want to live your life to its fullest potential, you need to find focus, discipline, and practice a tremendous amount of self discipline. The good news is by simply using the clear cut instructions and tips in this book, you can get quick, effective, and powerful results. I wish you nothing but the best success.

I really want to help you achieve your goals, and if you read this book and do the exercises for the next 30 days, I'm sure that you'll develop the focus and concentration you need to achieve your goals.

If you have a project that you need help with, email me at razasimam@outlook.com and I'll personally do what I can to help you get on track.

Please Leave a Review – It's Means a Lot

I hope you enjoyed this book. If you did, please leave me a review. It will only take 30 seconds and it would mean a LOT to me as an author.

We live and die by reviews:

- They help us know how our readers feel about our work
- They give us the motivation to keep writing
- They help others learn about our books

So please leave a review now.

Thanks in advance!

Made in the USA
Columbia, SC
21 July 2019